Daily Fitness and Nutrition Journal

Boston   Burr Ridge, IL   Dubuque, IA   Madison, WI   New York
San Francisco   St. Louis   Bangkok   Bogotá   Caracas   Kuala Lumpur
Lisbon   London   Madrid   Mexico City   Milan   Montreal   New Delhi
Santiago   Seoul   Singapore   Sydney   Taipei   Toronto

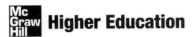

Higher Education

Daily Fitness and Nutrition Journal

1 2 3 4 5 6 7 8 9 0 FGR/FGR 0 9 8 7 6 5 4

ISBN 0-07-284432-9

www.mhhe.com

CONTENTS

FITNESS

Physical activity and exercise are key components of a wellness lifestyle. To live a long and healthy life, you must be active. The first part of this journal will help you develop a personalized plan for your fitness program. Once you are ready to put your plan into action, use the logs for weight training and for an overall exercise program to monitor the progress of your behavior change program.

First Steps

Before you begin to plan your fitness program, you should make sure that exercise is safe for you. If you are male and under 40 or female and under 50 and in good health, exercise is probably safe for you. If you are over these ages or have health problems, see your physician before starting an exercise program.

In addition, make sure that you are ready and motivated to increase your level of activity. Below, list the benefits and costs (pros and cons) of becoming more active and beginning a fitness program; include both short-term and long-term effects. Study your lists carefully. If you don't feel that the benefits of activity outweigh the costs, you'll have a more difficult time sticking with your program.

Benefits of increased physical activity:

_____

_____

_____

_____

_____

Costs of increased physical activity:

_____

_____

_____

_____

_____

Overall Program Plan

1. *Determine your current fitness status and activity level.* Below, briefly describe your current fitness status and activity level. What types of physical activity do you currently engage in? At what intensity and for how long? If you've performed formal fitness testing as part of a wellness or health course, include a summary of the results below.

Description of current activity/exercise habits:

_____

_____

_____

_____

_____

_____

_____

Results of fitness tests (test name and results):

_____

_____

_____

_____

_____

_____

_____

Are you satisfied with your current activity and fitness levels? Why or why not?

_____

_____

_____

_____

_____

_____

_____

2. *Set goals.* Based on your analysis of the costs and benefits of fitness and your current activity and fitness levels, set goals for your fitness program. Your goals can be specific or general, short or long term. In the first section, include specific, measurable goals that you can use to track the progress of your fitness program. These goals might be things like raising your cardiorespiratory fitness rating or swimming laps for 30 minutes without resting. In the second section, include long-term and more qualitative goals, such as improving the fit of your clothes and reducing your risk for chronic disease.

For each of your specific fitness goals, include a reward for achieving the goal. Rewards should be special, inexpensive, and preferably unrelated to food or alcohol.

Specific fitness goals:
   1. Current status: _____ Goal: _____
      Target date: _____ Reward: _____
   2. Current status: _____ Goal: _____
      Target date: _____ Reward: _____
   3. Current status: _____ Goal: _____
      Target date: _____ Reward: _____
   4. Current status: _____ Goal: _____
      Target date: _____ Reward: _____
   5. Current status: _____ Goal: _____
      Target date: _____ Reward: _____

General goals:
   1. _____
   2. _____
   3. _____
   4. _____
   5. _____

3. *Select activities.* Your program should be based around cardiorespiratory endurance exercise, but it should include activities that will develop all the different components of fitness. For example, your program might include bicycling, weight training, and stretching. Fill in the activities you've chosen on the overall program plan on the next page and check the components that each activity will develop.

    For weight training and stretching programs, you will need to select specific exercises to strengthen and stretch the different muscles of the body. Turn the page and fill in the exercises you've chosen for the weight training and stretching program plans. For each exercise in your weight training program, select a starting weight and number of repetitions and sets; add these to the "Weight Training Program Plan."

4. *Apply the FIT principle by setting a target frequency, intensity, and time for each activity.* Add these to the program plan on the next page. For advice on choosing activities and for determining appropriate frequency, intensity, and time (duration), refer to your textbook, visit the Web site of the American College of Sports Medicine (www.acsm.org), or consult an appropriate fitness professional.

5. *Begin and monitor your program.* Use the logs provided here to monitor your progress (see the weight training logs on pp. 8–23 and the overall fitness program logs on pp. 24–25). Be sure to complete the built-in progress check-ups every 6 weeks. To further track changes in your fitness status, record your starting resting heart rate (taken after 10 minutes of complete rest) in beats per minute and your blood pressure.

    Date: _____

    Resting heart rate: _____ bpm   Blood pressure: ____/____

Fitness Plan

Overall Program Plan

Activities	Components (Check ✔)					Frequency (Check ✔)							Intensity*	Time (Duration)
	Cardiorespiratory Endurance	Muscular Strength	Muscular Endurance	Flexibility	Body Composition	Monday	Tuesday	Wednesday	Thursday	Friday	Saturday	Sunday		
1.														
2.														
3.														
4.														
5.														
6.														

*You should conduct activities for achieving CRE goals at your target heart rate or RPE value.

5

Weight Training Program Plan

Exercise	Muscle(s) developed	Weight (lb)	Repetitions	Sets

Stretching Program Plan

Exercise	Area(s) stretched

Weight Training Logs

Exercise/Date								
	Wt							
	Sets							
	Reps							
	Wt							
	Sets							
	Reps							
	Wt							
	Sets							
	Reps							
	Wt							
	Sets							
	Reps							
	Wt							
	Sets							
	Reps							
	Wt							
	Sets							
	Reps							
	Wt							
	Sets							
	Reps							
	Wt							
	Sets							
	Reps							
	Wt							
	Sets							
	Reps							
	Wt							
	Sets							
	Reps							
	Wt							
	Sets							
	Reps							
	Wt							
	Sets							
	Reps							

Wt											
Sets											
Reps											
Wt											
Sets											
Reps											
Wt											
Sets											
Reps											
Wt											
Sets											
Reps											
Wt											
Sets											
Reps											
Wt											
Sets											
Reps											
Wt											
Sets											
Reps											
Wt											
Sets											
Reps											
Wt											
Sets											
Reps											
Wt											
Sets											
Reps											
Wt											
Sets											
Reps											
Wt											
Sets											
Reps											

Exercise/Date									
	Wt								
	Sets								
	Reps								
	Wt								
	Sets								
	Reps								
	Wt								
	Sets								
	Reps								
	Wt								
	Sets								
	Reps								
	Wt								
	Sets								
	Reps								
	Wt								
	Sets								
	Reps								
	Wt								
	Sets								
	Reps								
	Wt								
	Sets								
	Reps								
	Wt								
	Sets								
	Reps								
	Wt								
	Sets								
	Reps								
	Wt								
	Sets								
	Reps								
	Wt								
	Sets								
	Reps								

Wt													
Sets													
Reps													
Wt													
Sets													
Reps													
Wt													
Sets													
Reps													
Wt													
Sets													
Reps													
Wt													
Sets													
Reps													
Wt													
Sets													
Reps													
Wt													
Sets													
Reps													
Wt													
Sets													
Reps													
Wt													
Sets													
Reps													
Wt													
Sets													
Reps													
Wt													
Sets													
Reps													
Wt													
Sets													
Reps													

Weight Training

Exercise/Date									
	Wt								
	Sets								
	Reps								
	Wt								
	Sets								
	Reps								
	Wt								
	Sets								
	Reps								
	Wt								
	Sets								
	Reps								
	Wt								
	Sets								
	Reps								
	Wt								
	Sets								
	Reps								
	Wt								
	Sets								
	Reps								
	Wt								
	Sets								
	Reps								
	Wt								
	Sets								
	Reps								
	Wt								
	Sets								
	Reps								
	Wt								
	Sets								
	Reps								
	Wt								
	Sets								
	Reps								

Wt													
Sets													
Reps													
Wt													
Sets													
Reps													
Wt													
Sets													
Reps													
Wt													
Sets													
Reps													
Wt													
Sets													
Reps													
Wt													
Sets													
Reps													
Wt													
Sets													
Reps													
Wt													
Sets													
Reps													
Wt													
Sets													
Reps													
Wt													
Sets													
Reps													
Wt													
Sets													
Reps													

Weight Training

Exercise/Date									
	Wt								
	Sets								
	Reps								
	Wt								
	Sets								
	Reps								
	Wt								
	Sets								
	Reps								
	Wt								
	Sets								
	Reps								
	Wt								
	Sets								
	Reps								
	Wt								
	Sets								
	Reps								
	Wt								
	Sets								
	Reps								
	Wt								
	Sets								
	Reps								
	Wt								
	Sets								
	Reps								
	Wt								
	Sets								
	Reps								
	Wt								
	Sets								
	Reps								
	Wt								
	Sets								
	Reps								

Wt												
Sets												
Reps												
Wt												
Sets												
Reps												
Wt												
Sets												
Reps												
Wt												
Sets												
Reps												
Wt												
Sets												
Reps												
Wt												
Sets												
Reps												
Wt												
Sets												
Reps												
Wt												
Sets												
Reps												
Wt												
Sets												
Reps												
Wt												
Sets												
Reps												
Wt												
Sets												
Reps												

Exercise/Date								
	Wt							
	Sets							
	Reps							
	Wt							
	Sets							
	Reps							
	Wt							
	Sets							
	Reps							
	Wt							
	Sets							
	Reps							
	Wt							
	Sets							
	Reps							
	Wt							
	Sets							
	Reps							
	Wt							
	Sets							
	Reps							
	Wt							
	Sets							
	Reps							
	Wt							
	Sets							
	Reps							
	Wt							
	Sets							
	Reps							
	Wt							
	Sets							
	Reps							
	Wt							
	Sets							
	Reps							

Wt													
Sets													
Reps													
Wt													
Sets													
Reps													
Wt													
Sets													
Reps													
Wt													
Sets													
Reps													
Wt													
Sets													
Reps													
Wt													
Sets													
Reps													
Wt													
Sets													
Reps													
Wt													
Sets													
Reps													
Wt													
Sets													
Reps													
Wt													
Sets													
Reps													
Wt													
Sets													
Reps													
Wt													
Sets													
Reps													

Weight Training

Exercise/Date									
	Wt								
	Sets								
	Reps								
	Wt								
	Sets								
	Reps								
	Wt								
	Sets								
	Reps								
	Wt								
	Sets								
	Reps								
	Wt								
	Sets								
	Reps								
	Wt								
	Sets								
	Reps								
	Wt								
	Sets								
	Reps								
	Wt								
	Sets								
	Reps								
	Wt								
	Sets								
	Reps								
	Wt								
	Sets								
	Reps								
	Wt								
	Sets								
	Reps								
	Wt								
	Sets								
	Reps								

Wt													
Sets													
Reps													
Wt													
Sets													
Reps													
Wt													
Sets													
Reps													
Wt													
Sets													
Reps													
Wt													
Sets													
Reps													
Wt													
Sets													
Reps													
Wt													
Sets													
Reps													
Wt													
Sets													
Reps													
Wt													
Sets													
Reps													
Wt													
Sets													
Reps													
Wt													
Sets													
Reps													

Weight Training

Exercise/Date									
	Wt								
	Sets								
	Reps								
	Wt								
	Sets								
	Reps								
	Wt								
	Sets								
	Reps								
	Wt								
	Sets								
	Reps								
	Wt								
	Sets								
	Reps								
	Wt								
	Sets								
	Reps								
	Wt								
	Sets								
	Reps								
	Wt								
	Sets								
	Reps								
	Wt								
	Sets								
	Reps								
	Wt								
	Sets								
	Reps								
	Wt								
	Sets								
	Reps								
	Wt								
	Sets								
	Reps								
	Wt								
	Sets								
	Reps								

Wt												
Sets												
Reps												
Wt												
Sets												
Reps												
Wt												
Sets												
Reps												
Wt												
Sets												
Reps												
Wt												
Sets												
Reps												
Wt												
Sets												
Reps												
Wt												
Sets												
Reps												
Wt												
Sets												
Reps												
Wt												
Sets												
Reps												
Wt												
Sets												
Reps												
Wt												
Sets												
Reps												
Wt												
Sets												
Reps												

Exercise/Date									
	Wt								
	Sets								
	Reps								
	Wt								
	Sets								
	Reps								
	Wt								
	Sets								
	Reps								
	Wt								
	Sets								
	Reps								
	Wt								
	Sets								
	Reps								
	Wt								
	Sets								
	Reps								
	Wt								
	Sets								
	Reps								
	Wt								
	Sets								
	Reps								
	Wt								
	Sets								
	Reps								
	Wt								
	Sets								
	Reps								
	Wt								
	Sets								
	Reps								
	Wt								
	Sets								
	Reps								

Wt												
Sets												
Reps												
Wt												
Sets												
Reps												
Wt												
Sets												
Reps												
Wt												
Sets												
Reps												
Wt												
Sets												
Reps												
Wt												
Sets												
Reps												
Wt												
Sets												
Reps												
Wt												
Sets												
Reps												
Wt												
Sets												
Reps												
Wt												
Sets												
Reps												
Wt												
Sets												
Reps												
Wt												
Sets												
Reps												

Weight Training

Overall Fitness Program Logs

To use the overall fitness program logs, fill in the activities that are part of your program. Each day, note the distance and/or time you complete for each activity. For flexibility or weight training workouts, you may prefer just to enter a check mark each time you complete a workout. At the end of each week, total your distances and/or times.

SAMPLE

Date ____Oct 18–24____

Activity	M	Tu	W	Th	F	Sa	Su	Weekly Total
1. Walking (time)	30	40	30	45				145 min
2. Weight training	✔		✔		✔			3 days
3. Stretching		✔		✔		✔		3 days
4. Swimming (yards)						800		800 yards
5.								
6.								

Fitness Program

24

Date _____

Activity	M	Tu	W	Th	F	Sa	Su	Weekly Total
1.								
2.								
3.								
4.								
5.								
6.								

Date _____

Activity	M	Tu	W	Th	F	Sa	Su	Weekly Total
1.								
2.								
3.								
4.								
5.								
6.								

Date _____

Activity	M	Tu	W	Th	F	Sa	Su	Weekly Total
1.								
2.								
3.								
4.								
5.								
6.								

Date _____

Activity	M	Tu	W	Th	F	Sa	Su	Weekly Total
1.								
2.								
3.								
4.								
5.								
6.								

Date _____

Activity	M	Tu	W	Th	F	Sa	Su	Weekly Total
1.								
2.								
3.								
4.								
5.								
6.								

Date _____

Activity	M	Tu	W	Th	F	Sa	Su	Weekly Total
1.								
2.								
3.								
4.								
5.								
6.								

Fitness Program

Progress Check-Up: Week 6 of Program

Goals: Original Status   Current Status

_____   _____

_____   _____

_____   _____

_____   _____

_____   _____

Resting heart rate: _____ bpm Blood pressure: ____/____

Below, list the activities in your program, and describe how satisfied you are with each activity and with your overall progress. List any problems you've encountered or any unexpected costs or benefits of your fitness program so far.

Activity: _____ Status: _____

_____

Activity: _____ Status: _____

_____

Activity: _____ Status: _____

_____

Activity: _____ Status: _____

_____

What is your overall response to your program so far? How do you feel about your program and its effects?

Date _____

Activity	M	Tu	W	Th	F	Sa	Su	Weekly Total
1.								
2.								
3.								
4.								
5.								
6.								

Fitness Program

Date _____

Activity	M	Tu	W	Th	F	Sa	Su	Weekly Total
1.								
2.								
3.								
4.								
5.								
6.								

Date _____

Activity	M	Tu	W	Th	F	Sa	Su	Weekly Total
1.								
2.								
3.								
4.								
5.								
6.								

Date _____

Activity	M	Tu	W	Th	F	Sa	Su	Weekly Total
1.								
2.								
3.								
4.								
5.								
6.								

Date _____

Activity	M	Tu	W	Th	F	Sa	Su	Weekly Total
1.								
2.								
3.								
4.								
5.								
6.								

Date _____

Activity	M	Tu	W	Th	F	Sa	Su	Weekly Total
1.								
2.								
3.								
4.								
5.								
6.								

Progress Check-Up: Week 12 of Program

Goals: Original Status   Current Status

_____   _____

_____   _____

_____   _____

_____   _____

_____   _____

Resting heart rate: _____ bpm   Blood pressure: ____/____

Below, list the activities in your program, and describe how satisfied you are with each activity and with your overall progress. List any problems you've encountered or any unexpected costs or benefits of your fitness program so far.

Activity: _____   Status: _____
_____

Activity: _____   Status: _____
_____

Activity: _____   Status: _____
_____

Activity: _____   Status: _____
_____

What is your overall response to your program so far? How do you feel about your program and its effects?

Date _____

Activity	M	Tu	W	Th	F	Sa	Su	Weekly Total
1.								
2.								
3.								
4.								
5.								
6.								

Date _____

Activity	M	Tu	W	Th	F	Sa	Su	Weekly Total
1.								
2.								
3.								
4.								
5.								
6.								

Date _____

Activity	M	Tu	W	Th	F	Sa	Su	Weekly Total
1.								
2.								
3.								
4.								
5.								
6.								

Date _____

Activity	M	Tu	W	Th	F	Sa	Su	Weekly Total
1.								
2.								
3.								
4.								
5.								
6.								

Date _____

Activity	M	Tu	W	Th	F	Sa	Su	Weekly Total
1.								
2.								
3.								
4.								
5.								
6.								

Fitness Program

Date _____

Activity	M	Tu	W	Th	F	Sa	Su	Weekly Total
1.								
2.								
3.								
4.								
5.								
6.								

Progress Check-Up: Week 18 of Program

Goals: Original Status   Current Status

Original Status	Current Status
_____	_____
_____	_____
_____	_____
_____	_____
_____	_____

Resting heart rate: _____ bpm   Blood pressure: ____/____

Below, list the activities in your program, and describe how satisfied you are with each activity and with your overall progress. List any problems you've encountered or any unexpected costs or benefits of your fitness program so far.

Activity: _____   Status: _____

Activity: _____   Status: _____

Activity: _____   Status: _____

Activity: _____   Status: _____

What is your overall response to your program so far? How do you feel about your program and its effects?

Fitness Program

Date _____

Activity	M	Tu	W	Th	F	Sa	Su	Weekly Total
1.								
2.								
3.								
4.								
5.								
6.								

Date _____

Activity	M	Tu	W	Th	F	Sa	Su	Weekly Total
1.								
2.								
3.								
4.								
5.								
6.								

Date _____

Activity	M	Tu	W	Th	F	Sa	Su	Weekly Total
1.								
2.								
3.								
4.								
5.								
6.								

Date _____

Activity	M	Tu	W	Th	F	Sa	Su	Weekly Total
1.								
2.								
3.								
4.								
5.								
6.								

Date _____

Activity	M	Tu	W	Th	F	Sa	Su	Weekly Total
1.								
2.								
3.								
4.								
5.								
6.								

Date _____

Activity	M	Tu	W	Th	F	Sa	Su	Weekly Total
1.								
2.								
3.								
4.								
5.								
6.								

Progress Check-Up: Week 24 of Program

Goals: Original Status	Current Status
_____	_____
_____	_____
_____	_____
_____	_____
_____	_____

Resting heart rate: _____ bpm   Blood pressure: ____/____

Below, list the activities in your program, and describe how satisfied you are with each activity and with your overall progress. List any problems you've encountered or any unexpected costs or benefits of your fitness program so far.

Activity: _____ Status: _____
_____

Activity: _____ Status: _____
_____

Activity: _____ Status: _____
_____

Activity: _____ Status: _____
_____

What is your overall response to your program so far? How do you feel about your program and its effects?

Date _____

Activity	M	Tu	W	Th	F	Sa	Su	Weekly Total
1.								
2.								
3.								
4.								
5.								
6.								

Date _____

Activity	M	Tu	W	Th	F	Sa	Su	Weekly Total
1.								
2.								
3.								
4.								
5.								
6.								

Date _____

Activity	M	Tu	W	Th	F	Sa	Su	Weekly Total
1.								
2.								
3.								
4.								
5.								
6.								

Date _____

Activity	M	Tu	W	Th	F	Sa	Su	Weekly Total
1.								
2.								
3.								
4.								
5.								
6.								

Date _____

Activity	M	Tu	W	Th	F	Sa	Su	Weekly Total
1.								
2.								
3.								
4.								
5.								
6.								

Date _____

Activity	M	Tu	W	Th	F	Sa	Su	Weekly Total
1.								
2.								
3.								
4.								
5.								
6.								

Progress Check-Up: Week 30 of Program

Goals: Original Status   Current Status

_____   _____

_____   _____

_____   _____

_____   _____

_____   _____

Resting heart rate: _____ bpm   Blood pressure: ___/___

Below, list the activities in your program, and describe how satisfied you are with each activity and with your overall progress. List any problems you've encountered or any unexpected costs or benefits of your fitness program so far.

Activity: _____   Status: _____

Activity: _____   Status: _____

Activity: _____   Status: _____

Activity: _____   Status: _____

What is your overall response to your program so far? How do you feel about your program and its effects?

Fitness Program

Date _____

Activity	M	Tu	W	Th	F	Sa	Su	Weekly Total
1.								
2.								
3.								
4.								
5.								
6.								

Date _____

Activity	M	Tu	W	Th	F	Sa	Su	Weekly Total
1.								
2.								
3.								
4.								
5.								
6.								

Date _____

Activity	M	Tu	W	Th	F	Sa	Su	Weekly Total
1.								
2.								
3.								
4.								
5.								
6.								

Date _____

Activity	M	Tu	W	Th	F	Sa	Su	Weekly Total
1.								
2.								
3.								
4.								
5.								
6.								

Date _____

Activity	M	Tu	W	Th	F	Sa	Su	Weekly Total
1.								
2.								
3.								
4.								
5.								
6.								

Date _____

Activity	M	Tu	W	Th	F	Sa	Su	Weekly Total
1.								
2.								
3.								
4.								
5.								
6.								

Progress Check-Up: Week 36 of Program

Goals: Original Status   Current Status

_____   _____

_____   _____

_____   _____

_____   _____

_____   _____

Resting heart rate: _____ bpm Blood pressure: ____/____

Below, list the activities in your program, and describe how satisfied you are with each activity and with your overall progress. List any problems you've encountered or any unexpected costs or benefits of your fitness program so far.

Activity: _____ Status: _____

_____

Activity: _____ Status: _____

_____

Activity: _____ Status: _____

_____

Activity: _____ Status: _____

_____

What is your overall response to your program so far? How do you feel about your program and its effects?

Date _____

Activity	M	Tu	W	Th	F	Sa	Su	Weekly Total
1.								
2.								
3.								
4.								
5.								
6.								

Date _____

Activity	M	Tu	W	Th	F	Sa	Su	Weekly Total
1.								
2.								
3.								
4.								
5.								
6.								

Date _____

Activity	M	Tu	W	Th	F	Sa	Su	Weekly Total
1.								
2.								
3.								
4.								
5.								
6.								

Date _____

Activity	M	Tu	W	Th	F	Sa	Su	Weekly Total
1.								
2.								
3.								
4.								
5.								
6.								

Date _____

Activity	M	Tu	W	Th	F	Sa	Su	Weekly Total
1.								
2.								
3.								
4.								
5.								
6.								

Date _____

Activity	M	Tu	W	Th	F	Sa	Su	Weekly Total
1.								
2.								
3.								
4.								
5.								
6.								

Progress Check-Up: Week 42 of Program

Goals: Original Status   Current Status

_____   _____

_____   _____

_____   _____

_____   _____

_____   _____

Resting heart rate: _____ bpm Blood pressure: ____/____

Below, list the activities in your program, and describe how satisfied you are with each activity and with your overall progress. List any problems you've encountered or any unexpected costs or benefits of your fitness program so far.

Activity: _____ Status: _____

Activity: _____ Status: _____

Activity: _____ Status: _____

Activity: _____ Status: _____

What is your overall response to your program so far? How do you feel about your program and its effects? Do you think you will stick with your program? Why or why not?

NUTRITION

Nutrition is a vitally important component of wellness. Diet influences energy levels, well-being, and overall health. A well-planned diet supports maximum fitness and protects against disease. This part of your journal will help you analyze your current eating habits, identify patterns that may be causing you to shortchange yourself on nutrition, and put a more balanced eating plan into action.

To start monitoring, assessing, and improving your nutritional habits, follow these steps:

1. Review the tools for keeping a nutrition log provided on pages 54–60.
2. Using these tools, fill out the Preprogram Nutrition Log for 3 days.
3. Use the Assessing Your Daily Diet worksheets to analyze your daily nutritional intake. Do you see some areas in your current diet that could be improved?
4. Complete the Behavior Change Contract. The information in the Tools for Improving Your Food Choices section will help you identify unhealthy behaviors and plan how to improve them.
5. Record your daily diet a second time in the Postprogram Nutrition Log.
6. Analyze your revised diet and compare it to your original diet.

Once you understand your nutritional needs and habits, you can make reasonable and healthy choices for weight management. Additional nutrition log pages are provided for longer term monitoring of your diet.

Nutrition

TOOLS FOR MONITORING YOUR DAILY DIET

The Food Guide Pyramid

Use the Food Guide Pyramid as a guide to daily food choices. The Pyramid is an outline of what to eat each day—not a rigid prescription, but a general guide that lets you choose a healthful diet that's right for you. It calls for eating a variety of foods to get the nutrients you need and at the same time the right amount of calories to maintain a healthy weight.

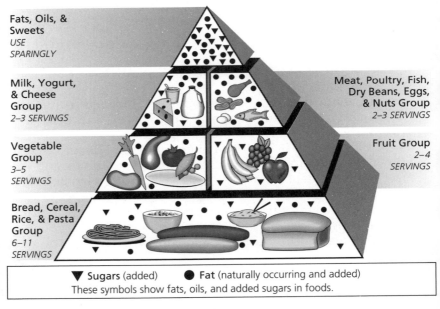

Fats, Oils, & Sweets
USE SPARINGLY

Milk, Yogurt, & Cheese Group
2–3 SERVINGS

Meat, Poultry, Fish, Dry Beans, Eggs, & Nuts Group
2–3 SERVINGS

Vegetable Group
3–5 SERVINGS

Fruit Group
2–4 SERVINGS

Bread, Cereal, Rice, & Pasta Group
6–11 SERVINGS

▼ **Sugars** (added)   ● **Fat** (naturally occurring and added)
These symbols show fats, oils, and added sugars in foods.

Figure 1. The Food Guide Pyramid

Source: Center for Nutrition Policy and Information. 1996. *Food Guide Pyramid*. USDA, Home and Garden Bulletin No. 252.

Food Groups and Recommended Servings

The recommendations of the Pyramid are based on serving sizes. Refer to this table for the recommended number of servings and some examples of serving sizes for each group:

Food Group	Number of Servings	Foods and Serving Sizes
Milk, yogurt, and cheese	2–3	1 cup milk $1^1/_2$ oz cheese 2 oz processed cheese 1 cup yogurt
Meat, poultry, fish, dry beans, eggs, and nuts	2–3*	2–3 oz cooked meat, poultry, fish 1–$1^1/_2$ cups cooked dry beans 4 tbsp peanut butter 2 eggs $^1/_2$–1 cup nuts
Fruits	2–4	1 medium or 2 small whole fruit(s) 1 melon wedge $^1/_2$ cup berries $^1/_2$ grapefruit $^1/_4$ cup dried fruit $^1/_2$ cup cooked or canned fruit $^3/_4$ cup juice (100% juice)
Vegetables	3–5	$^1/_2$ cup raw or cooked vegetables 1 cup raw leafy vegetables $^3/_4$ cup juice
Bread, cereals, rice, and pasta	6–11	1 slice of bread $^1/_2$ hamburger bun, English muffin, or bagel (depending on size) 1 small roll, biscuit, or muffin 1 oz ready-to-eat cereal $^1/_2$ cup cooked cereal, rice, or pasta 5–6 small or 2–3 large crackers
Fats, oils, and sweets		Foods from this group should not replace any from the other groups. Amounts consumed should be determined by individual energy needs.

*Your total daily intake should be the equivalent of 5–7 ounces of cooked lean meat, poultry, or fish. The following portions of nonmeat foods are equivalent to 1 ounce of lean meat: 1 egg, 2 tbsp peanut butter, $^1/_3$ cup nuts, $^1/_4$ cup seeds, $^1/_2$ cup tofu.

When you use the table on the previous page to determine the number of servings you should be eating from each food group, remember that the range of servings is designed to accommodate a range of calorie levels depending on age, gender, and level of activity. The low end of the recommended range of servings is about right for many sedentary women and older adults; the middle of the range is about right for most children, teenage girls, active women, and many sedentary men; and the top of the range is about right for teenage boys, many active men, and some very active women.

Making Choices Within the Food Groups

As shown in the Food Groups and Recommended Servings table, you can choose from a variety of foods in each food group to fulfill your daily needs. The average American diet is at or below the low end of the servings range for most food groups, but we eat too much fat and added sugars to meet the recommendations without gaining weight. The key is to make better food choices within the groups and so get more nutrients for your calories. Keep these guidelines in mind as you plan your meals:

General

- Choose a variety of foods within each group. Different foods contain different combinations of nutrients.
- If you are concerned about eating too much and gaining weight, concentrate on nutrient-dense foods— foods that are high in nutrients relative to the amount of calories they contain.

Milk, yogurt, and cheese

- Pick nonfat milk and yogurt over whole milk and regular yogurt.
- Choose "part skim" or low-fat cheeses, ice milk, and frozen yogurt over their higher-fat counterparts.
- If you are trying to increase your calcium consumption, remember that cottage cheese is lower in calcium than many other dairy products.

Meat, poultry, fish, dry beans, eggs, and nuts

- The choices lowest in fat in this group are lean meat, skinless poultry, fish, and dry beans and peas.
- Trim the fat from meat and prepare it by broiling, roasting, or boiling.
- Use egg yolks, nuts, and seeds in moderation.

Fruits

- Choose fresh fruits, fruit juices, and frozen, canned, or dried fruit over fruit in heavy syrups or sweetened fruit drinks.
- To increase your fiber intake, choose whole fruits over fruit juices.
- Choose citrus fruit, melons, and berries for the most vitamin C.

Vegetables

- To take advantage of the different nutrients found in various types of vegetables, include servings of each type in your diet regularly: dark-green leafy vegetables, deep-yellow vegetables, starchy vegetables, legumes, and other vegetables.
- Choose dark-green leafy vegetables and legumes often; they are especially rich in vitamins and minerals.

Bread, cereals, rice, and pasta

- For a healthy fiber and nutrient intake, have several servings a day of foods made from whole grains.
- Choose most often foods in this group with little fat or sugar, such as bread, rice, and pasta.
- Limit your consumption of baked goods included in this group but high in fat and sugar such as cakes, cookies, croissants, and pastries.
- Try preparing packaged pasta, stuffing, and sauces using half the butter suggested or low-fat milk in place of milk or cream.

Nutrition

Self-Assessment: Portion Size Quiz

Now test yourself to see if your perception of serving sizes is the same as those used with the Food Guide Pyramid (check your answers on the next page). Remember that when you keep your nutrition log you will need to assess your intake using the Pyramid serving sizes.

1. An ounce and a half of hard cheese—equivalent to one serving from the dairy group—looks most like
   a. one domino.
   b. two dominoes.
   c. three dominoes.

2. A half cup of cooked pasta, considered a serving from the grain group, most easily fits into
   a. an ice cream scoop (the kind with a release handle).
   b. a ball the size of a medium grapefruit.
   c. a cereal bowl.

3. One drink of wine roughly fills
   a. two-thirds of a coffee cup.
   b. one coffee cup.
   c. two coffee cups.

4. One serving of green grapes consists of how many grapes?
   a. 10
   b. 15
   c. 20

5. Three ounces of beef, a serving's worth, most closely resembles
   a. a *T.V. Guide.*
   b. a regular bar of soap.
   c. a small bar of soap (as from a hotel).

6. One serving of brussels sprouts consists of how many sprouts?
   a. 4
   b. 8
   c. 12

7. Two tablespoons of olive oil more or less fill
   a. a shot glass.
   b. a thimble.
   c. a Dixie cup.

8. Two tablespoons of peanut butter make a ball the size of
   a. a marble.
   b. a tennis ball.
   c. a Ping-Pong ball.

9. How many shakes of a five-hole salt shaker does it take to reach 1 teaspoon (approximately the maximum amount of salt recommended per day)?
   a. 5
   b. 10
   c. 60

10. There are eight servings in a loaf of Entenmann's Raspberry Danish Twist. A serving is the width of
    a. one finger.
    b. two fingers.
    c. four fingers.

Answers

1. c	3. a	5. b	7. a	9. c
2. a	4. b	6. a	8. c	10. b

Source: What's in a Portion? *Tufts University Diet and Nutrition Letter,* September, 1994. Reprinted with permission, *Tufts University Health and Nutrition Letter* (1-800-274-7581).

Reading Food Labels

Another important tool for keeping your nutrition log is the information you will find on food labels. In the example on page 60, note that the serving size is 1 cup. If you eat 2 cups of chili, you'll need to double all the values on the label. Other useful information includes total calories and calories from fat per serving. Remember that the serving size given on the food label is often not the same as the serving size specified by the Food Guide Pyramid, and neither one may be the size of the serving you choose for yourself.

Nutrition

1. Serving size: Determine how many servings there are in the food package and compare it to how much you actually eat. You may need to adjust the rest of the nutrient values based on your typical serving size.

2. Calories and calories from fat: Note whether a serving is high in calories and fat. The sample food shown here is low in fat, with only 30 of its 235 calories from fat.

3. Daily Values: Based on a 2000-calorie diet, Daily Value percentages tell you whether the nutrients in a serving of food contribute a lot or a little to your total daily diet.
> **5% or less is low**
> **20% or more is high**

4. Limit these nutrients: Look for foods low in fat, saturated fat, trans fat, cholesterol, and sodium. *(Trans fat content must be included on the label by January 2006 for any food with more than 0.5g trans fat per serving.)*

5. Get enough of these nutrients: Look for foods high in dietary fiber, vitamin A, vitamin C, calcium, and iron.

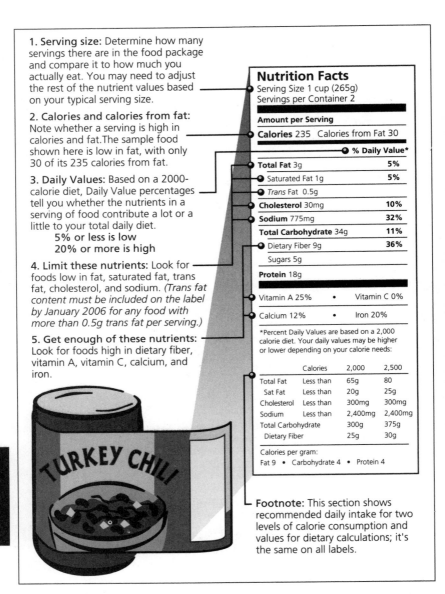

Nutrition Facts
Serving Size 1 cup (265g)
Servings per Container 2

Amount per Serving

Calories 235   Calories from Fat 30

	% Daily Value*
Total Fat 3g	**5%**
Saturated Fat 1g	**5%**
Trans Fat 0.5g	
Cholesterol 30mg	**10%**
Sodium 775mg	**32%**
Total Carbohydrate 34g	**11%**
Dietary Fiber 9g	**36%**
Sugars 5g	
Protein 18g	

Vitamin A 25%	•	Vitamin C 0%
Calcium 12%	•	Iron 20%

*Percent Daily Values are based on a 2,000 calorie diet. Your daily values may be higher or lower depending on your calorie needs:

	Calories	2,000	2,500
Total Fat	Less than	65g	80
Sat Fat	Less than	20g	25g
Cholesterol	Less than	300mg	300mg
Sodium	Less than	2,400mg	2,400mg
Total Carbohydrate		300g	375g
Dietary Fiber		25g	30g

Calories per gram:
Fat 9 • Carbohydrate 4 • Protein 4

Footnote: This section shows recommended daily intake for two levels of calorie consumption and values for dietary calculations; it's the same on all labels.

TURKEY CHILI

Figure 2. Food Label

Nutrition

PREPROGRAM NUTRITION LOG

Keep a record of everything you eat for 3 consecutive days. Record all foods and beverages you consume, breaking each food item into its component parts (for example, a turkey sandwich would be listed as 2 slices of bread, 3 oz of turkey, 1 tsp of mayonnaise, and so on). Complete the first two columns of the chart, indicating the food that you ate and the portion size, during the course of the day. At the end of the day, fill in the food group and number of servings for everything that you consumed, using the Food Guide Pyramid, the table of food groups and recommended servings, information from food labels, and the appendix at the end of this journal listing the nutritional content of items from fast-food restaurants.

Nutrition

Preprogram Nutrition Log

DAY 1

Food	Portion Size	Food Group	Number of Servings*

*Your portion sizes may be smaller or larger than the serving sizes given in the Food Guide Pyramid; list the actual number of Food Guide Pyramid servings contained in the foods you eat.

Preprogram Nutrition Log

DAY 2

Food	Portion Size	Food Group	Number of Servings*

*Your portion sizes may be smaller or larger than the serving sizes given in the Food Guide Pyramid; list the actual number of Food Guide Pyramid servings contained in the foods you eat.

Nutrition

Preprogram Nutrition Log

DAY 3

Food	Portion Size	Food Group	Number of Servings*

*Your portion sizes may be smaller or larger than the serving sizes given in the Food Guide Pyramid; list the actual number of Food Guide Pyramid servings contained in the foods you eat.

ASSESSING YOUR DAILY DIET

A balanced diet follows the Food Guide Pyramid recommendations. Fill in the actual number of servings from each food group that you recorded, and compare them to the recommended number of servings.

DAY 1 TOTAL

Food Group	Recommended Servings	Actual Servings
Milk, yogurt, cheese	2–3	
Meat, poultry, fish, dry beans, eggs, nuts	2–3	
Fruits	2–4	
Vegetables	3–5	
Breads, cereals, rice, pasta	6–11	
Fats, oils, sweets	use sparingly	

DAY 2 TOTAL

Food Group	Recommended Servings	Actual Servings
Milk, yogurt, cheese	2–3	
Meat, poultry, fish, dry beans, eggs, nuts	2–3	
Fruits	2–4	
Vegetables	3–5	
Breads, cereals, rice, pasta	6–11	
Fats, oils, sweets	use sparingly	

DAY 3 TOTAL

Food Group	Recommended Servings	Actual Servings
Milk, yogurt, cheese	2–3	
Meat, poultry, fish, dry beans, eggs, nuts	2–3	
Fruits	2–4	
Vegetables	3–5	
Breads, cereals, rice, pasta	6–11	
Fats, oils, sweets	use sparingly	

Nutrition

NUTRITION BEHAVIOR CHANGE CONTRACT

Have you identified some areas of your diet where you don't meet the Food Guide Pyramid recommendations? Perhaps you have more than the recommended servings of meat in your diet or don't eat enough vegetables. Take a good look at your current diet and think about the changes you can make to improve it. Use the Behavior Change Contract on the next page to record your plan for dietary change and the steps that you will follow to reach your goal.

1. Fill in your name and your target for change. Examples of behavior change targets include increasing daily servings of vegetables and decreasing servings of sweets.

2. Enter a start date, final goal, and target completion date. Allow enough time to achieve your overall goal. Make your goal specific, such as increasing fruit intake from 2 servings per week to 2 servings per day.

3. Break your program into several stages and give yourself a reward for achieving each mini-goal in addition to a reward for reaching your final goal.

4. List specific strategies for achieving your goal, including such things as packing fruit in your backpack every morning, getting up 15 minutes earlier to allow time for a sit-down breakfast, and stocking your refrigerator with healthy beverages. Your program will probably involve making trade-offs: Review your nutrition logs and identify foods high in fat and sugar and low in other nutrients; these are foods to target for reduction or elimination. For additional tips, go to the Tools for Improving Your Food Choices section and use the quizzes and tables there (pp. 68–72).

5. Use the logs provided in this journal or develop your own plan for monitoring your eating habits and the progress of your program.

6. Sign your contract and, if possible, recruit a witness who can also participate in your program. (Your helper might eat a meal with you each day or call to offer encouragement.)

Behavior Change Contract

1. I _____ agree to
_____

2. I will begin on _____ and plan to reach my
goal of _____ by _____

3. In order to reach my final goal, I have devised the following
schedule of mini-goals. For each step in my program, I will give
myself the reward listed:

Mini-goal	Target date	Reward
_____	_____	_____
_____	_____	_____
_____	_____	_____

My overall reward for reaching my final goal will be
_____

4. My plan for reaching my goal includes the following strategies:
_____
_____
_____
_____
_____

5. I will use the following tools to monitor my progress toward
reaching my final goal:
_____
_____

I sign this contract as an indication of my personal commitment
to reach my goal.

Your signature: _____ Date: _____

I have recruited a helper who will witness my contract and
_____
_____

Witness signature: _____ Date: _____

67

TOOLS FOR IMPROVING YOUR FOOD CHOICES

Dietary Guidelines for Americans

As you plan to change your diet, keep in mind the Dietary Guidelines for Americans. These guidelines, which are described in more detail in your textbook and at the Web site for the USDA Center for Nutrition Policy and Promotion (www.usda.gov/cnpp), provide a good foundation for a lifestyle that promotes health. They are organized under three messages, the "ABCs for Health":

- **A**im for fitness

  Aim for a healthy weight

  Be physically active each day

- **B**uild a healthy base

  Let the Pyramid guide your food choices

  Choose a variety of grains daily, especially whole grains

  Choose a variety of fruits and vegetables daily

  Keep food safe to eat

- **C**hoose sensibly

  Choose a diet that is low in saturated fat and cholesterol and moderate in total fat

  Choose beverages and foods to moderate your intake of sugars

  Choose and prepare foods with less salt

  If you drink alcoholic beverages, do so in moderation

Making Healthy Ethnic Food Choices

	Choose Often	Choose Seldom
Chinese	Chinese Greens Hunan or Szechuan dishes Rice, brown or white Steamed dishes Stir-fry dishes Wonton soup	Crispy duck or beef Egg rolls or fried wontons General Tso's chicken Kung pao dishes Rice, fried Sweet-and-sour dishes
Italian	Cioppino (seafood stew) Minestrone soup, vegetarian Pasta with marinara sauce Pasta primavera Pasta with red or white clam sauce	Cannelloni, ravioli, or manicotti Fettucini alfredo Fried calamari Garlic bread Veal or eggplant parmigiana
Indian	Chapati (baked tortilla-like bread) Dal (lentils) Karhi (chick-pea soup) Khur (milk and rice dessert) Tandoori, chicken or fish Yogurt-based curry dishes	Bhatura, poori, or paratha (fried breads) Coconut milk-based dishes Ghee (clarified butter) Korma (rich meat dish) Pakoras (fried appetizer) Samosa (fried meat and vegetables in dough)
Japanese	Kushiyaki (broiled foods on skewers) Shabu-shabu (foods in boiling broth) Sushi	Agemono (deep-fried foods) Sukiyaki Tonkatsu (fried pork) Tempura (fried chicken, shrimp, or vegetables)

Nutrition

	Choose Often	**Choose Seldom**
Mexican	Beans and rice	Chiles relleños
	Black bean and vegetable soup	Chimichangas or flautas
	Burritos, bean or chicken	Enchiladas, beef or cheese
	Fajitas, chicken or vegetable	Nachos or fried tortillas
	Gazpacho	Quesadillas
	Refried beans, nonfat or low-fat	Refried beans made with lard
	Tortillas, steamed	Taco salad
Thai	Forest salad	Fried fish, duck, or chicken
	Larb (chicken salad with mint)	Curries with coconut milk
	Po tak (seafood stew)	Dishes with peanut sauce
	Yum neua (broiled beef with onions)	Yum koon chaing (sausage with peppers)

Source: The sat fat switch; 1997. *Nutrition Action Healthletter,* January/February. University of Southern Florida University of Southern Florida Student Health Service. 1997. Ethnic food (http://www.shs/usf.edu/Health/ethnic.html). The best of Asian cuisines, 1993; *University of California at Berkeley Wellness Letter,* January. Eating in ethnic restaurants, 1990; *Runner's World,* January. Reprinted by permission of *Runner's World Magazine.*

Self-Assessment: What Triggers Your Eating?

Hunger isn't the only reason people eat. Efforts to make healthy eating choices can be sabotaged by eating related to other factors, such as emotions or patterns of thinking. Your score on this quiz will help you understand your motivations for eating so that you can create an effective plan for changing your eating behavior. Circle the number that indicates to what degree each situation is likely to make you start eating.

Social

	Very Unlikely	Very Likely
1. Arguing or being in conflict with someone	1 2 3 4 5	6 7 8 9 10
2. Being with others when they are eating	1 2 3 4 5	6 7 8 9 10
3. Being urged to eat by someone else	1 2 3 4 5	6 7 8 9 10

Social (continued)

4. Feeling inadequate
   around others
   1 2 3 4 5 6 7 8 9 10

Emotional

5. Feeling bad, such as
   being anxious or depressed
   1 2 3 4 5 6 7 8 9 10

6. Feeling good, happy,
   or relaxed
   1 2 3 4 5 6 7 8 9 10

7. Feeling bored or having
   time on my hands
   1 2 3 4 5 6 7 8 9 10

8. Feeling stressed or excited
   1 2 3 4 5 6 7 8 9 10

Situational

9. Seeing an advertisement
   for food or eating
   1 2 3 4 5 6 7 8 9 10

10. Passing by a bakery,
    cookie shop, or other
    enticement to eat
    1 2 3 4 5 6 7 8 9 10

11. Being involved in a
    party, celebration, or
    special occasion
    1 2 3 4 5 6 7 8 9 10

12. Eating out
    1 2 3 4 5 6 7 8 9 10

Thinking

13. Making excuses to
    myself about why it's
    okay to eat
    1 2 3 4 5 6 7 8 9 10

14. Berating myself for
    being so fat or unable
    to control my eating
    1 2 3 4 5 6 7 8 9 10

15. Worrying about others or
    about difficulties I am having
    1 2 3 4 5 6 7 8 9 10

16. Thinking about
    how things should or
    shouldn't be
    1 2 3 4 5 6 7 8 9 10

Physiological

17. Experiencing pain
    or discomfort
    1 2 3 4 5 6 7 8 9 10

Nutrition

Physiological (continued)	Very Unlikely							Very Likely		
18. Experiencing trembling, headache, or lightheadedness associated with no eating or too much caffeine	1	2	3	4	5	6	7	8	9	10
19. Experiencing fatigue or feeling overtired	1	2	3	4	5	6	7	8	9	10
20. Experiencing hunger pangs or urges to eat, even though I've eaten recently	1	2	3	4	5	6	7	8	9	10

Scoring

Total your scores for each area and enter them below. Then rank the scores by marking the highest score "1," next highest score "2," and so on. Focus on the highest-ranked areas first, but any score above 24 is high and indicates that you need to work on that area.

Area	Total Score	Rank Score
Social (Items 1–4)	_____	_____
Emotional (Items 5–8)	_____	_____
Situational (Items 9–12)	_____	_____
Thinking (Items 13–16)	_____	_____
Physiological (Items 17–20)	_____	_____

Lowering a High Score

Social Try reducing your susceptibility to the influence of others by communicating more assertively and rethinking your beliefs about obligations you feel you must fulfill.

Emotional Develop stress-management skills and practice positive self-talk to cope with emotions in ways that don't involve food.

Situational Work on controlling your environment and having a plan for handling external cues.

Thinking Change your thinking—be less self-critical and more flexible—to recognize rationalizations and excuses about eating behavior.

Physiological Look at the way you eat, what you eat, and medications to find ways these factors may be affecting your eating behavior.

Source: What Triggers Your Eating? Adapted from Nash, J. D. 1997. *The New Maximize Your Body Potential*. Palo Alto, Calif: Bull Publishing. Reprinted with permission from Bull Publishing Company.

Nutrition

POSTPROGRAM NUTRITION LOG

Now that you have analyzed your diet and targeted some changes described in your Behavior Change Contract, you are ready to put your plan into action. Fill out this second nutrition log, again keeping a record of everything you eat for 3 consecutive days. Remember to record all foods and beverages you consume, breaking each food item into its component parts (for example, a turkey sandwich would be listed as 2 slices of bread, 3 oz of turkey, 1 tsp of mayonnaise, and so on). Complete the first two columns of the chart, indicating the food that you ate and the portion size, during the course of the day. At the end of the day, fill in the food group and number of servings for everything that you consumed, using the Food Guide Pyramid, the food groups and recommended servings table, information from food labels, and the appendix listing the nutritional content of items from fast-food restaurants.

Nutrition

Postprogram Nutrition Log

DAY 1

Food	Portion Size	Food Group	Number of Servings*

*Your portion sizes may be smaller or larger than the serving sizes given in the Food Guide Pyramid; list the actual number of Food Guide Pyramid servings contained in the foods you eat.

Postprogram Nutrition Log

DAY 2

Food	Portion Size	Food Group	Number of Servings*

*Your portion sizes may be smaller or larger than the serving sizes given in the Food Guide Pyramid; list the actual number of Food Guide Pyramid servings contained in the foods you eat.

Nutrition

Postprogram Nutrition Log

DAY 3

Food	Portion Size	Food Group	Number of Servings*

*Your portion sizes may be smaller or larger than the serving sizes given in the Food Guide Pyramid; list the actual number of Food Guide Pyramid servings contained in the foods you eat.

ASSESSING IMPROVEMENT IN YOUR DAILY DIET

Fill in the actual number of servings from each food group that you recorded in your Postprogram Nutrition Log, and compare them to the recommended number of servings. To check the progress you have made, transfer the results from the Preprogram Nutrition Log and compare them to the results of your new diet.

DAY 1 TOTAL

Food Group	Recommended Servings	Actual Servings	Preprogram Servings
Milk, yogurt, cheese	2–3		
Meat, poultry, fish, dry beans, eggs, nuts	2–3		
Fruits	2–4		
Vegetables	3–5		
Breads, cereals, rice, pasta	6–11		
Fats, oils, sweets	use sparingly		

DAY 2 TOTAL

Food Group	Recommended Servings	Actual Servings	Preprogram Servings
Milk, yogurt, cheese	2–3		
Meat, poultry, fish, dry beans, eggs, nuts	2–3		
Fruits	2–4		
Vegetables	3–5		
Breads, cereals, rice, pasta	6–11		
Fats, oils, sweets	use sparingly		

Nutrition

DAY 3 TOTAL

Food Group	Recommended Servings	Actual Servings	Preprogram Servings
Milk, yogurt, cheese	2–3		
Meat, poultry, fish, dry beans, eggs, nuts	2–3		
Fruits	2–4		
Vegetables	3–5		
Breads, cereals, rice, pasta	6–11		
Fats, oils, sweets	use sparingly		

In comparing the results of my postprogram log to the results of my preprogram log, I found that

_____

_____

Completing a Behavior Change Contract and following its steps helped me to

_____

_____

Areas of improvement that I will focus on in the future are

_____

_____

_____

_____

You can use the additional logs that follow (pp. 79–85) to track your diet in the future; for tips on weight management, go to p. 86.

Nutrition Log

Date _____

Food	Portion Size	Food Group	Number of Servings*

*Your portion sizes may be smaller or larger than the serving sizes given in the Food Guide Pyramid; list the actual number of Food Guide Pyramid servings contained in the foods you eat.

Nutrition

Nutrition Log

Date _____

Food	Portion Size	Food Group	Number of Servings*

*Your portion sizes may be smaller or larger than the serving sizes given in the Food Guide Pyramid; list the actual number of Food Guide Pyramid servings contained in the foods you eat.

Nutrition Log

Date _____

Food	Portion Size	Food Group	Number of Servings*

*Your portion sizes may be smaller or larger than the serving sizes given in the Food Guide Pyramid; list the actual number of Food Guide Pyramid servings contained in the foods you eat.

Nutrition

Nutrition Log

Date _____

Food	Portion Size	Food Group	Number of Servings*

*Your portion sizes may be smaller or larger than the serving sizes given in the Food Guide Pyramid; list the actual number of Food Guide Pyramid servings contained in the foods you eat.

Nutrition

Nutrition Log

Date _____

Food	Portion Size	Food Group	Number of Servings*

*Your portion sizes may be smaller or larger than the serving sizes given in the Food Guide Pyramid; list the actual number of Food Guide Pyramid servings contained in the foods you eat.

Nutrition

Nutrition Log

Date _____

Food	Portion Size	Food Group	Number of Servings*

*Your portion sizes may be smaller or larger than the serving sizes given in the Food Guide Pyramid; list the actual number of Food Guide Pyramid servings contained in the foods you eat.

Nutrition Log

Date _____

Food	Portion Size	Food Group	Number of Servings*

*Your portion sizes may be smaller or larger than the serving sizes given in the Food Guide Pyramid; list the actual number of Food Guide Pyramid servings contained in the foods you eat.

WEIGHT MANAGEMENT

CREATING A WEIGHT MANAGEMENT PROGRAM

Completing the preprogram and postprogram nutrition logs will help you monitor and improve your daily diet. If you decide that your weight or percent body fat is above or below the amount that is appropriate for your size, gender, and age, the information you have gathered with your nutrition logs will be an important part of a weight management program. This section outlines the general steps in a weight management program; in the next section you'll track activity and food choices to identify ways to create a negative energy balance and lose weight.

Follow these steps to develop your weight management program and put it into action:

1. Assess Your Motivation and Commitment

Make sure you are motivated and committed to your plan for weight management before you begin. It is important to understand why you want to change your weight or body composition. You will generally be more successful if your reasons are self-focused, such as wanting to feel good about yourself, rather than connected to others' perceptions of you.

When you understand your reasons for wanting to manage your weight, list them below. Post your list in a prominent place as a reminder.

1. _____

2. _____

3. _____

4. _____

2. Set Goals

After you have chosen a reasonable long-term weight or body-fat percentage goal, break your progress into a series of short-term goals. You can include a small, non-food-related reward like a new CD or a night at the movies for successfully reaching each goal.

	Goal	Reward
1.	_____	_____
2.	_____	_____
3.	_____	_____
4.	_____	_____

3. Assess Your Current Energy Balance

When your weight is stable, you are burning approximately the same number of calories that you are taking in. In order to lose weight, you must consume fewer calories, burn more calories through physical activity, or both. This will create a negative energy balance that will lead to gradual, moderate weight loss. Strategies for creating a negative energy balance are discussed on page 89 of this journal.

4. Increase Your Level of Physical Activity

You can increase your energy output simply by increasing your routine physical activity, such as walking or taking the stairs. You will increase your energy output even more if you adopt a program of regular exercise like the one described in the first section of this journal.

5. Evaluate Your Diet and Eating Habits

Take another look at the nutrition logs you completed. Are there some high-calorie, low-nutrient foods that stand out? If your increase in physical activity does not result in a negative energy balance that produces weight loss, you may want to make small cuts in your calorie intake by reducing your consumption of these foods.

Weight Management

6. Track Your Physical Activity and Diet

Use the weight management logs to record your daily physical activities and dietary choices. These logs will help you un-cover potential calorie savings that will create a negative calorie balance and help you lose weight.

For People Who Want to Gain Weight

If the goal of your weight management program is to increase your weight, you'll need to create a positive energy balance by taking in more calories than you use. The basis of a success-ful and healthy program for weight gain is a combination of strength training and a high-calorie diet. Strength training will help you add weight as muscle rather than as fat. To increase your calorie consumption, eat more high-carbohydrate foods, including grains, vegetables, and fruits. (Fatty, high-calorie foods may seem like a logical choice for weight gain, but a diet high in fat carries health risks, and your body is likely to convert dietary fat into body fat rather than into muscle.) Avoid skipping meals, add two or three snacks to your daily diet, and consider adding a dietary supplement high in carbo-hydrates, protein, vitamins, and minerals. As with weight loss, a gradual program of weight gain is the best strategy.

CREATING A NEGATIVE ENERGY BALANCE

A reasonable weight-loss goal is ½–1 pound per week. Depending on your individual characteristics, you will need to create a negative energy balance of between 1750 and 3500 calories a week, or 250–500 calories a day. While this may seem daunting, you already make choices every day that affect your energy balance significantly. Making a few decisions each day with your energy balance in mind can add up to a successful weight management program.

First, review the sample weight management log on the next page that shows the daily activities of Elizabeth, a hypothetical 21-year-old student weighing 130 pounds. As she goes through her day, she has many opportunities to make choices that will affect her energy balance. In the real world, you will be more likely to make one or two choices each day that decrease the number of calories you take in or increase the number of calories you expend. The key is to be aware of your opportunities to affect your energy balance and to make healthy choices as often as possible without making yourself feel deprived.

After you have reviewed this example, record and assess your own daily choices using the blank weight management logs that follow. Fill in your activities and your meals and snacks, and then think about alternatives you could have chosen. What would the potential calorie savings have been if you had made these choices? To calculate the calories you expended in physical activity, consult the table of common sports and fitness activities on page 90 of this journal, information in your text, and materials on energy balance in the report from the Surgeon General on physical activity and the Surgeon General's Call to Action on obesity (available online at www.surgeongeneral.gov). To calculate calories saved by making a healthier food choice, use information in your text, the fast food data available at the back of this journal, and the USDA online nutrient database (www.nal.usda.gov/fnic/cgi-bin/nut_search.pl).

Weight Management

CALORIE COSTS FOR COMMON SPORTS AND FITNESS ACTIVITIES

When you change your energy balance by participating in an activity that expends calories, how do you calculate how many calories you have actually spent? Calorie costs are given here for 10 common activities; use these as benchmarks for calculating the calorie costs of other activities.

Multiply the number in the appropriate column (moderate or vigorous) by your body weight and then by the number of minutes you exercise. (If you participate in your activity at a level between moderate and vigorous, use a number between the two values.) For example, if you weigh 150 pounds and play tennis vigorously for 45 minutes, multiply .071 (value) by 150 (weight) and then by 45 (time) for a result of 479 calories expended.

| | **Approximate Calorie Cost** | |
Activity	*Moderate*	*Vigorous*
Aerobic dance	.046	.062
Basketball, half court	.045	.071
Bicycling	.049	.071
Hiking	.051	.073
Jogging and running	.060	.104
Racquetball, skilled, singles	.049	.078
Skating, ice, roller, and in-line	.049	.095
Swimming	.032	.088
Tennis, skilled, singles	—	.071
Walking	.029	.048

Sample Daily Weight Management Log

Activity/Meal or Snack	Healthier Choice (describe)	Approximate Calorie Savings
Friday morning, Elizabeth eats breakfast: a croissant and a cup of coffee with cream.	Friday morning, Elizabeth eats breakfast: a bowl of whole-grain cereal, a glass of orange juice, and a cup of coffee. She uses most of a glass of skim milk for her cereal and puts the rest in her coffee.	81
Elizabeth drives to campus.	Elizabeth walks 15 minutes to campus.	57
After class, Elizabeth visits her friend's dorm, where they watch the noon soap opera for an hour.	After class, Elizabeth meets her friend for a 25-minute jog.	195
For lunch, Elizabeth eats 2 slices of leftover pepperoni pizza and drinks a soda.	After their jog, they have lunch at the dorm; each has a turkey sandwich, an apple, and iced tea.	231
Elizabeth goes to her afternoon class. She wants a snack, so she buys a candy bar from the vending machine.	Elizabeth goes to her afternoon class. She wants a snack, so she buys a nonfat yogurt with fruit in the student union.	142
Elizabeth drives home.	Elizabeth walks 15 minutes home.	57
Elizabeth studies until her roommates get home.	Elizabeth studies until her roommates get home.	—
Elizabeth and her roommates decide to stop for fast food on the way to the movies. Elizabeth orders a cheeseburger, large french fries, and a small chocolate shake.	Elizabeth and her roommates decide to stop for fast food on the way to the movies. Elizabeth orders a hamburger, a green salad with carrots and fat-free dressing, and a small chocolate shake.	389
At the movies, Elizabeth shares a bag of buttered popcorn with her friend.	At the movies, Elizabeth shares a bag of air-popped popcorn with her friend.	64

Daily Weight Management Log

Activity/Meal or Snack	Healthier Choice (describe)	Approximate Calorie Savings

Daily Weight Management Log

Activity/Meal or Snack	Healthier Choice (describe)	Approximate Calorie Savings

Daily Weight Management Log

Activity/Meal or Snack	Healthier Choice (describe)	Approximate Calorie Savings

Daily Weight Management Log

Activity/Meal or Snack	Healthier Choice (describe)	Approximate Calorie Savings

Weight Management

Daily Weight Management Log

Activity/Meal or Snack	Healthier Choice (describe)	Approximate Calorie Savings

Weight Management

Daily Weight Management Log

Activity/Meal or Snack	Healthier Choice (describe)	Approximate Calorie Savings

Daily Weight Management Log

Activity/Meal or Snack	Healthier Choice (describe)	Approximate Calorie Savings

Daily Weight Management Log

Activity/Meal or Snack	Healthier Choice (describe)	Approximate Calorie Savings

Weight Management

Daily Weight Management Log

Activity/Meal or Snack	Healthier Choice (describe)	Approximate Calorie Savings

Weight Management

APPENDIX Nutritional Content of Popular Items from Fast-Food Restaurants

Arby's

	Serving size	Calories	Protein	Total fat	Saturated fat	Total Carbohydrate	Sugars	Fiber	Cholesterol	Sodium	Vitamin A	Vitamin C	Calcium	Iron	% Calories from fat
	g		g	g	g	g	g	g	mg	mg	% RDI	% RDI	% RDI	% RDI	
Regular roast beef	157	350	21	16	6	34	N/A	2	85	950	N/A	0	6	20	41
Super roast beef	245	470	22	23	7	47	N/A	3	85	1130	N/A	2	8	20	44
French dip	285	440	28	18	8	42	N/A	2	100	1680	N/A	2	8	25	37
Junior roast beef	129	310	16	13	4.5	34	N/A	2	70	740	N/A	0	6	15	38
Roast chicken Caesar sandwich	363	820	43	38	9	75	N/A	5	140	2160	N/A	15	35	25	42
Roast turkey & Swiss	360	760	43	33	6	75	N/A	5	130	1920	N/A	4	35	25	39
Chicken breast fillet	208	540	24	30	5	47	N/A	2	90	1160	N/A	6	8	10	50
Hot ham 'n Swiss sandwich	170	340	23	13	4.5	35	N/A	1	90	1450	N/A	2	15	15	34
Jalapeño bites™	111	330	7	21	9	30	N/A	2	40	670	N/A	2	4	4	57
Cheddar curly fries	170	460	6	24	6	54	N/A	4	5	1290	N/A	25	6	10	47
Potato cakes (2)	100	250	2	16	4	26	N/A	3	0	490	N/A	10	0	4	58
Grilled chicken Caesar salad	338	230	33	8	3.5	8	N/A	3	80	920	N/A	70	20	10	31
Thousand Island dressing	57	290	1	28	4.5	9	N/A	0	35	480	N/A	0	0	0	87
French-toastix	124	370	7	17	4	48	N/A	4	0	440	N/A	0	7	10	41

N/A: not available.

SOURCE: Arby's © 2004, Arby's, Inc. (http://www.arbysrestaurant.com). Used with permission of Arby's, Inc. Nutritional information contained in this Arby's, Inc. brochure was obtained from independent lab analysis, Genesis Nutrition and Diet Software, supplier information, and the USDA Handbook #8. Information on Arby's products contained herein is based on laboratory and calculated analysis of Arby's ingredients as of April 2004. Actual nutritional information may differ based on regional variability in product availability and in individual unit compliance with Arby's Standard Operating Procedures. Information is not to be used by individuals with special dietary needs in lieu of professional medical advice.

Burger King

	Serving size (g)	Calories	Protein (g)	Total fat (g)	Saturated fat (g)	Trans fat (g)	Total Carbohydrate (g)	Sugars (g)	Fiber (g)	Cholesterol (mg)	Sodium (mg)	Vitamin A	Vitamin C	Calcium	Iron	% Calories from fat
												% Daily Value				
Original WHOPPER®	291	700	31	42	13	1	52	8	4	85	1020	20	15	10	30	54
Original WHOPPER® w/o mayo	270	540	30	24	10	1	52	8	4	75	900	10	15	10	30	40
Original DOUBLE WHOPPER® w/cheese	399	1060	56	69	27	3	53	9	4	185	1540	25	15	30	45	59
Original WHOPPER JR.®	158	390	17	22	7	0.5	31	5	2	45	550	10	6	8	15	51
BK VEGGIE® Burger*	186	380	14	16	2.5	0	46	6	4	5	930	15	6	8	35	38
Chicken WHOPPER®	272	570	38	25	4.5	0	48	5	4	75	1410	15	10	6	40	39
CHICKEN TENDERS® (8 pieces)	123	340	22	19	5	3.5	20	0	<1	50	840	2	2	2	4	50
French fries (medium, salted)	117	360	4	18	5	4.5	46	1	4	0	640	0	2	2	4	45
Onion rings (medium)	91	320	4	16	4	3.5	40	5	3	0	460	0	10	10	0	45
Chili (w/o cheese or crackers)	217	190	13	8	3	0	17	5	5	25	1040	25	8	8	8	38
Fire-grilled chicken caesar salad (w/o dressing or toast)	286	190	25	7	3	0	9	1	1	50	900	80	40	15	8	33
CROISSAN'WICH® w/bacon, egg, and cheese	119	360	15	22	8	2	25	4	<1	195	950	8	0	30	20	55
HERSHEY®'S sundae pie	79	300	3	18	10	1.5	31	23	1	10	190	2	0	4	6	54
Chocolate Shake (medium)	397	600	10	18	11	2	97	94	2	70	470	15	6	45	8	27

* Burger King Corporation makes no claim that the BK VEGGIE® Burger or any of its products meets the requirements of a vegan or vegetarian diet.

SOURCE: BURGER KING® nutritional information used with permission from Burger King Brands, Inc.

102

Domino's Pizza

(1 serving = 2 of 8 slices or ¼ of 14-inch pizza; 2 of 8 slices or ¼ of 12-inch pizza; 1 6-inch pizza)

	Serving size	Calories	Protein	Total fat	Saturated fat	Total carbohydrate	Sugars	Fiber	Cholesterol	Sodium	Vitamin A	Vitamin C	Calcium	Iron	% calories from fat
	g	g	g	g	g	g	g	g	mg	mg	% Daily Value				
14-inch lg. hand-tossed cheese	219	516	21	15	7	75	6	4	32	1080	18	0	26	23	26
14-inch lg. thin crust cheese	148	382	17	17	7	43	6	2	32	1172	18	0	32	8	40
14-inch lg. deep dish cheese	256	677	26	30	11	80	9	5	41	1575	21	<1	33	31	40
12-inch med. hand-tossed cheese	159	375	15	11	5	55	5	3	23	776	13	0	19	17	26
12-inch med. thin crust cheese	106	273	12	12	5	31	4	2	23	835	13	0	23	5	40
12-inch med. deep dish cheese	181	482	19	22	8	56	6	3	30	1123	15	<1	24	22	41
Toppings: pepperoni	*	98	5	9	3	<1	<1	<1	20	364	<1	<1	<1	2	83
ham	*	31	5	2	<1	<1	<1	<1	12	292	<1	<1	<1	1	58
Italian sausage	*	110	5	9	3	3	<1	<1	22	342	<1	2	2	3	74
bacon	*	153	8	13	4	<1	<1	<1	22	424	0	15	<1	2	77
beef	*	111	6	10	4	<1	<1	<1	21	309	<1	0	<1	3	81
anchovies	*	45	9	2	<1	<1	<1	<1	18	791	<1	0	5	6	40
extra cheese	*	68	6	6	3	<1	<1	<1	15	228	6	0	12	<1	79
cheddar cheese	*	71	6	6	3	<1	<1	<1	18	110	4	0	13	<1	76
Barbeque buffalo wings (1 piece)	25	50	6	2	<1	2	1	<1	26	175	<1	<1	<1	2	36
Buffalo chicken kickers™ (1 piece)	24	47	4	2	<1	3	<1	<1	9	163	<1	<1	<1	0	38
Blue cheese sauce	42	223	1	23	4	2	2	<1	20	417	1	2	2	<1	93
Breadsticks (1 stick)	37	116	3	4	<1	18	1	1	0	152	<1	<1	<1	5	31
Double cheesy bread	43	142	4	6	2	18	1	1	6	183	2	<1	5	5	38

* Topping information is based on minimal portioning requirements for one serving of a 14-inch large pizza; add the values for toppings to the values for a cheese pizza. The following toppings supply fewer than 15 calories per serving: green and yellow peppers, onion, olives, mushrooms, pineapple.

SOURCE: Domino's Pizza, 2004 (http://www.dominos.com). Reproduced with permission from Domino's Pizza LLC.

Jack in the Box

	Serving size (g)	Calories	Protein (g)	Total fat (g)	Saturated fat (g)	Total carbohydrate (g)	Sugars (g)	Fiber (g)	Cholesterol (mg)	Sodium (mg)	Vitamin A	Vitamin C	Calcium	Iron	% Calories from fat
											% Daily Value				
Breakfast Jack®	129	310	13	14	5	33	4	1	205	720	N/A	N/A	N/A	N/A	42
Supreme croissant	171	570	19	37	9	41	5	1	240	1040	N/A	N/A	N/A	N/A	58
Hamburger	119	310	17	14	6	30	6	1	45	600	N/A	N/A	N/A	N/A	42
Jumbo Jack® w/cheese	314	690	27	38	16	61	13	3	70	1360	N/A	N/A	N/A	N/A	49
Sourdough Jack®	244	700	30	49	16	36	7	3	80	1220	N/A	N/A	N/A	N/A	63
Chicken fajita pita	230	330	24	11	4.5	35	4	3	55	910	N/A	N/A	N/A	N/A	30
Sourdough grilled chicken club	249	520	33	28	6	33	5	3	85	1330	N/A	N/A	N/A	N/A	48
Ultimate club	316	640	37	30	9	51	7	3	105	2000	N/A	N/A	N/A	N/A	42
Jack's Spicy Chicken®	308	730	30	37	10	69	9	4	70	1480	N/A	N/A	N/A	N/A	45
Monster taco	119	260	9	15	5	21	4	3	30	340	N/A	N/A	N/A	N/A	50
Egg rolls (3)	170	400	14	19	6	44	4	6	15	920	N/A	N/A	N/A	N/A	43
Chicken breast pieces (5)	150	360	27	17	3	24	0	1	80	970	N/A	N/A	N/A	N/A	43
Stuffed jalapeños (7)	168	530	15	30	13	51	5	4	45	1600	N/A	N/A	N/A	N/A	51
Barbeque dipping sauce	28	45	0	0	0	11	4	0	0	330	N/A	N/A	N/A	N/A	0
Seasoned curly fries	125	400	6	23	5	45	1	5	0	890	N/A	N/A	N/A	N/A	52
Onion rings	119	500	6	30	5	51	3	3	0	420	N/A	N/A	N/A	N/A	54
Side salad	137	50	3	3	1.5	4	2	2	10	65	N/A	N/A	N/A	N/A	54
Thousand Island dressing	57	160	0	12	2	12	10	0	15	490	N/A	N/A	N/A	N/A	68
Oreo® cookie ice-cream shake (16 oz)	301	670	11	33	19	81	62	1	110	350	N/A	N/A	N/A	N/A	45

N/A: not available.

SOURCE: Jack in the Box, Inc. 2003 (http://www.jackinthebox.com). The following trademarks are owned by Jack in the Box, Inc.: Breakfast Jack,® Jumbo Jack,® Sourdough Jack,® Jack in the Box.® Reproduced with permission from Jack in the Box, Inc.

KFC

	Serving size (g)	Calories (g)	Protein (g)	Total fat (g)	Saturated fat (g)	Total Carbohydrate (g)	Sugars (g)	Fiber (g)	Cholesterol (mg)	Sodium (mg)	Vitamin A	Vitamin C	Calcium	Iron	% calories from fat
											% Daily Value				
Original Recipe® breast	161	380	40	19	6	11	0	0	145	1145	0	0	0	6	45
Original Recipe® thigh	126	360	22	25	7	12	0	0	165	1060	0	0	0	6	63
Extra Crispy™ breast	162	460	34	28	8	19	0	0	135	1230	0	0	0	8	55
Extra Crispy™ thigh	114	370	21	26	7	12	0	0	120	710	0	0	0	6	63
Hot & Spicy breast	179	460	33	27	8	20	0	0	130	1450	0	0	0	6	53
Hot & Spicy thigh	128	400	22	28	8	14	0	0	125	1240	0	0	0	8	63
Tender Roast® sandwich w/sauce	196	390	31	19	4	24	0	1	70	810	0	0	4	10	44
Tender Roast® sandwich w/o sauce	177	260	31	5	1.5	23	0	1	65	690	0	4	4	10	17
Hot Wings™ pieces (6)	134	450	24	29	6	23	1	1	145	1120	6	8	8	10	58
Colonel's Crispy Strips® (3)	151	400	29	24	5	17	1	0	75	1250	6	0	0	10	54
Popcorn chicken (large)	170	660	29	44	10	37	0	0	75	1530	0	4	4	35	60
Chicken pot pie	423	770	33	40	15	70	5	5	115	1680	200	0	0	20	47
Corn on the cob (5.5")	162	150	5	3	1	26	10	7	0	10	0	6	6	6	18
Mashed potatoes w/gravy	136	120	2	4.5	1	18	<1	1	0	380	2	0	2	2	34
BBQ baked beans	136	230	8	1	1	46	22	7	0	720	8	6	15	30	4
Cole slaw	130	190	1	11	2	22	13	3	5	300	25	40	4	0	52
Biscuit (1)	57	190	2	10	2	23	1	1	0	580	0	0	0	4	47
Potato salad	128	190	2	11	2	22	5	1	5	470	0	10	0	2	52

SOURCE: KFC Corporation, 2004 (http://www.kfc.com). Reproduced with permission from Kentucky Fried Chicken Corporation.

105

Subway

Based on standard formulas with
6-inch subs on Italian or wheat bread

	Serving size (g)	Calories	Protein (g)	Total fat (g)	Saturated fat (g)	Total carbohydrate (g)	Sugars (g)	Fiber (g)	Cholesterol (mg)	Sodium (mg)	Vitamin A	Vitamin C	Calcium	Iron	% calories from fat
											% Daily Value				
Italian BMT®	248	450	23	21	8	47	8	4	55	1790	10	35	15	20	42
Meatball Marinara	287	500	23	22	11	52	9	5	45	1180	10	40	15	35	40
Subway® Seafood Sensation	255	380	16	13	4.5	52	8	5	25	1170	10	35	15	20	31
Cheese steak	256	360	24	10	4.5	47	9	5	35	1090	10	35	15	40	25
Turkey breast, ham & bacon melt	260	380	25	12	5	47	8	4	45	1610	10	35	15	20	28
Classic tuna	255	430	20	19	5	46	7	5	45	1070	10	35	15	20	40
Sweet onion chicken teriyaki	266	370	26	5	1.5	58	18	4	50	1100	8	45	8	20	12
Honey mustard ham	243	310	19	5	1.5	54	14	5	25	1410	8	35	6	20	15
Roast beef	222	290	19	5	2	45	8	4	20	910	8	35	6	30	16
Turkey breast, ham & roast beef	255	320	24	6	2	47	8	4	35	1300	8	35	6	30	17
Savory turkey breast	222	280	18	4.5	1.5	46	7	4	20	1010	8	35	6	20	14
Veggie Delite®	166	230	9	3	1	44	7	4	0	510	8	35	6	20	12
Savory turkey breast deli	151	210	13	3.5	1.5	36	4	3	15	730	6	20	6	20	15
Chicken Bacon Ranch Wrap	215	480	40	27	9	19	3	11	95	1340	6	15	40	10	51
Bacon and egg breakfast sandwich	123	320	15	15	4.5	34	3	3	185	520	6	6	8	20	42
Garden fresh salad w/ Seafood Sensation (w/o dressing or toppings)	380	210	10	11	3.5	20	7	5	25	740	160	80	20	10	47
Garden fresh salad	300	60	3	1	0	11	5	5	0	80	160	80	8	10	15
New England clam chowder	240	110	5	3.5	0.5	16	1	1	10	990	2	10	10	0	29
Chili con carne	240	240	15	10	5	23	14	8	15	860	15	6	6	6	38
Sunrise refresher (small)	341	120	1	0	0	29	28	1	0	20	4	210	2	0	0
Choclate chip cookie	45	210	2	10	4	30	18	1	15	160	4	0	0	6	43

SOURCE: Subway U.S. Nutrition Info as found on http://www.subway.com, 4/23/2004. Reprented by permission of Subway.

Taco Bell

	Serving size (g)	Calories (g)	Protein (g)	Total fat (g)	Saturated fat (g)	Total Carbohydrate (g)	Sugars (g)	Fiber (g)	Cholesterol (mg)	Sodium (mg)	Vitamin A (% Daily Value)	Vitamin C (% Daily Value)	Calcium (% Daily Value)	Iron (% Daily Value)	% Calories from fat
Taco	78	170	8	10	4	13	1	3	25	350	6	4	6	6	53
Taco Supreme®	113	220	9	14	7	14	2	3	40	360	10	8	8	8	57
Soft taco, beef	99	210	10	10	4.5	21	2	2	25	620	6	4	10	10	43
Soft Taco Supreme,® chicken	134	230	15	10	5	21	3	1	45	570	8	8	15	6	39
Gordita Supreme,® steak	153	290	16	13	6	28	7	2	35	520	6	6	10	15	37
Gordita Baja,® chicken	153	320	17	15	3.5	29	7	2	40	690	6	6	10	10	42
Chalupa Supreme, beef	153	390	14	24	10	31	5	3	40	600	10	8	15	10	55
Chalupa Supreme, chicken	153	370	17	20	8	30	4	1	45	530	6	8	10	6	49
Bean burrito	198	370	14	10	3.5	55	4	8	10	1200	10	8	20	15	24
Burrito Supreme,® chicken	248	410	21	14	6	50	5	5	45	1270	15	15	20	15	31
Grilled stuffed burrito, beef	325	730	28	33	11	79	7	10	55	2080	20	10	35	25	41
Tostada	170	250	11	10	4	29	2	7	15	710	10	8	15	8	36
Zesty Chicken Border Bowl™ w/dressing	417	730	23	42	9	65	5	12	45	1640	20	15	15	20	52
Taco salad with salsa	533	790	31	42	15	73	10	13	65	1670	30	35	40	35	48
Steak quesadilla	184	540	26	31	14	40	4	3	70	1370	15	0	50	15	52
Nachos Supreme	195	450	13	26	9	42	4	7	35	800	8	10	10	10	58
Nachos BellGrande®	308	780	20	43	13	80	6	12	35	1300	10	10	20	15	50
Pintos 'n cheese	128	180	10	7	3.5	20	1	6	15	700	10	6	15	6	35
Mexican rice	131	210	6	10	4	23	<1	3	15	740	20	8	10	10	43

SOURCE: Taco Bell Corporation, 2003 (http://www.tacobell.com). Reproduced courtesy of Taco Bell Corporation.

Wendy's

	Serving size (g)	Calories	Protein (g)	Total fat (g)	Saturated fat (g)	Trans fat (g)	Total carbohydrate (g)	Sugars (g)	Fiber (g)	Cholesterol (mg)	Sodium (mg)	Vitamin A	Vitamin C	Calcium	Iron	% Calories from fat
												% Daily Value				
Classic Single® w/everything	218	410	25	19	7	1	37	8	2	70	910	N/A	N/A	N/A	N/A	42
Big Bacon Classic®	282	580	33	29	12	1.5	45	11	3	95	1430	N/A	N/A	N/A	N/A	45
Jr. hamburger	117	270	15	9	3.5	0.5	34	7	2	30	610	N/A	N/A	N/A	N/A	30
Jr. bacon cheeseburger	165	380	20	19	7	1	34	6	2	55	830	N/A	N/A	N/A	N/A	45
Ultimate Chicken Grill Sandwich	225	360	31	7	1.5	0	44	11	2	75	1100	N/A	N/A	N/A	N/A	18
Spicy Chicken Fillet Sandwich	225	510	29	19	3.5	1.5	57	8	2	55	1480	N/A	N/A	N/A	N/A	34
Homestyle Chicken Fillet Sandwich	230	540	29	22	4	1.5	57	2	2	55	1320	N/A	N/A	N/A	N/A	37
Caesar side salad (no toppings or dressing)	99	70	6	4.5	2	0	2	1	1	10	190	N/A	N/A	N/A	N/A	58
Chicken BLT salad (no toppings or dressing)	376	360	34	19	9	0.5	10	4	4	95	1140	N/A	N/A	N/A	N/A	48
Taco Supremo salad (no toppings or dressing)	495	360	27	16	8	1	29	8	8	65	1090	N/A	N/A	N/A	N/A	40
Creamy ranch dressing	64	230	1	23	4	0.5	5	3	0	15	580	N/A	N/A	N/A	N/A	90
Reduced fat creamy ranch dressing	64	100	1	8	1.5	0	6	3	1	15	550	N/A	N/A	N/A	N/A	72
Biggie® fries	159	440	5	19	3.5	5	63	0	7	0	380	N/A	N/A	N/A	N/A	39
Baked potato w/broccoli & cheese	411	440	10	15	3	0	70	6	9	10	540	N/A	N/A	N/A	N/A	31
Baked potato w/bacon & cheese	380	560	16	25	7	0	67	6	7	35	910	N/A	N/A	N/A	N/A	40
Chili, small, plain	227	200	17	5	2	0	21	5	5	35	870	N/A	N/A	N/A	N/A	23
Chili, large w/cheese	357	370	29	13	6.5	1.5	32	7	7	65	1420	N/A	N/A	N/A	N/A	32
Crispy Chicken Nuggets™ (5)	75	220	10	14	3	0	13	0	0	35	490	N/A	N/A	N/A	N/A	57
Barbecue sauce (1 packet)	28	40	1	0	0	0	10	5	0	0	160	N/A	N/A	N/A	N/A	0
Frosty,™ medium	298	430	10	11	7	0	74	55	0	45	200	N/A	N/A	N/A	N/A	23

SOURCE: Wendy's International, Inc., 2004 (http://www.wendys.com). Reproduced with permission from Wendy's International, Inc.

Information on additional foods and restaurants is available online; see the Web sites listed with the tables in this appendix and the following additional sites:

Hardees: http://www.hardees.com   McDonald's: http://www.mcdonalds.com   White Castle: http://www.whitecastle.com